I0410287

Barrett's Esophagus Guide for Beginners

Importance of Understanding Barrett's Esophagus

By

Guthrie Fintan
Copyright@2023

Table of Contents

CHAPTER 1

Introduction

Barrett's Esophagus is a condition that affects the lining of the lower esophagus, and it has garnered significant attention in the medical field due to its potential to progress into a more serious condition, specifically esophageal adenocarcinoma. This introduction will provide a detailed exploration of Barrett's Esophagus, encompassing its definition, a historical overview, and the critical importance of understanding this condition.

1.1 Definition of Barrett's Esophagus

Barrett's Esophagus, named after the Australian-born British surgeon Norman Barrett, is a chronic medical condition characterized by changes in the cells lining the lower part of the esophagus. Normally, the esophageal lining consists of squamous cells, but in individuals with Barrett's Esophagus, these cells are replaced by a specialized type of cell known as intestinal metaplasia. This transformation is largely attributed to chronic and severe gastroesophageal reflux disease (GERD) or acid reflux, where stomach acid frequently flows back into the esophagus.

One of the defining features of Barrett's Esophagus is its association with a heightened risk of developing esophageal adenocarcinoma, a type of cancer. While not everyone with Barrett's Esophagus will develop cancer, understanding this condition is of paramount importance because it serves as a precursor to a potentially life-threatening disease.

1.2 Historical Overview

Barrett's Esophagus was first described in medical literature by Dr. Norman Barrett in 1950. Dr. Barrett's pioneering work shed light on the distinct changes in the esophageal lining that occur in certain individuals. At that time, the condition was not widely recognized, and its clinical significance remained largely unknown.

Over the decades, advances in medical research and technology have allowed for a deeper understanding of

Barrett's Esophagus. This includes the development of endoscopic techniques that enable doctors to directly visualize and biopsy the esophagus, facilitating early diagnosis and monitoring of the condition. The historical perspective underscores the evolution of our knowledge about Barrett's Esophagus and the remarkable progress made in its diagnosis and management.

1.3 Importance of Understanding Barrett's Esophagus

Understanding Barrett's Esophagus is of paramount importance for several critical reasons:

1. **Cancer Risk:** Barrett's Esophagus is a significant risk

factor for the development of esophageal adenocarcinoma, one of the deadliest cancers. While not everyone with Barrett's Esophagus will develop cancer, it represents a precursor condition, and early detection and management can potentially prevent cancer from developing.

2. **Preventive Measures:** Recognizing the link between chronic GERD and Barrett's Esophagus underscores the importance of managing acid reflux and adopting preventive measures. Lifestyle modifications and appropriate medical interventions can reduce the risk of this condition.

3. **Early Detection:** Regular surveillance and screening of individuals with Barrett's Esophagus are essential for early detection of any dysplastic changes or progression to cancer. Timely intervention can significantly improve treatment outcomes.

4. **Treatment Strategies:** Understanding the condition enables healthcare providers to tailor treatment strategies to individual patients. Management may include lifestyle changes, medication, endoscopic therapy, or surgery, depending on the severity and progression of Barrett's Esophagus.

5. **Quality of Life:** Managing Barrett's Esophagus can lead to

improved quality of life for affected individuals. Effective management of GERD symptoms and monitoring of Barrett's Esophagus can reduce discomfort and complications associated with the condition.

Barrett's Esophagus is a condition with historical significance and contemporary medical relevance. It stands as a bridge between chronic acid reflux and esophageal adenocarcinoma, emphasizing the critical importance of early diagnosis, careful monitoring, and appropriate management. Understanding Barrett's Esophagus empowers individuals and healthcare providers to take proactive steps in safeguarding health and preventing the potential progression to a life-threatening disease.

CHAPTER 2

Causes and Risk Factors

Barrett's Esophagus is a complex medical condition influenced by various factors, both intrinsic and extrinsic. Understanding the causes and risk factors associated with Barrett's Esophagus is essential in comprehending its development and progression. In this extensive exploration, we delve into the key contributors to Barrett's Esophagus, encompassing Gastroesophageal Reflux Disease (GERD), genetics and family history, obesity and lifestyle factors, as well as other significant elements.

2.1 Gastroesophageal Reflux Disease (GERD)

Gastroesophageal Reflux Disease (GERD) stands out as the primary and most widely recognized risk factor for Barrett's Esophagus. GERD is a chronic condition in which stomach acid and, occasionally, stomach contents, flow back into the esophagus. This reflux occurs due to the weakening of the lower esophageal sphincter, a muscular ring that normally acts as a barrier to prevent the contents of the stomach from entering the esophagus.

The persistent exposure of the esophageal lining to stomach acid can lead to chronic inflammation and irritation. Over time, this can cause changes in the cells of the esophageal lining, ultimately resulting in Barrett's Esophagus. The esophagus attempts to protect itself from the acid by replacing its normal squamous cells with specialized intestinal cells, a process known as intestinal metaplasia.

The severity and duration of GERD symptoms are directly correlated with the risk of developing Barrett's Esophagus. Frequent and long-lasting symptoms, such as heartburn and regurgitation, increase the likelihood of esophageal damage and subsequent metaplasia.

2.2 Genetics and Family History

Genetics plays a significant role in the development of Barrett's Esophagus. Individuals with a family history of Barrett's Esophagus or esophageal cancer are at an increased risk. This suggests a hereditary component in the susceptibility to the condition. Research has identified certain genetic factors that may predispose individuals to Barrett's Esophagus, although the precise genes involved are still under investigation.

It is worth noting that while genetics can increase the risk, environmental factors, such as diet and lifestyle, also contribute substantially to the development of Barrett's Esophagus. Family history should be considered as just one piece of the puzzle in understanding an individual's risk.

2.3 Obesity and Lifestyle Factors

Obesity is another significant risk factor for Barrett's Esophagus. Excess body weight, particularly abdominal obesity, increases the pressure on the abdomen, which can force stomach acid into the esophagus. Additionally, fat tissue can produce hormones and chemicals that may contribute to inflammation and changes in the esophageal lining.

Lifestyle factors, such as diet and smoking, are also known contributors to Barrett's Esophagus. A diet high in fatty, fried, and acidic foods can exacerbate GERD symptoms, potentially leading to esophageal damage over time. Smoking, on the other hand, can weaken the lower esophageal sphincter and reduce the body's ability to clear stomach acid, both of which heighten the risk of Barrett's Esophagus.

Alcohol consumption is another lifestyle factor that can exacerbate GERD and increase the risk of Barrett's Esophagus. Alcohol can relax the lower esophageal sphincter, allowing acid to reflux into the esophagus more easily.

2.4 Other Contributing Factors

While GERD, genetics, obesity, and lifestyle factors are among the most prominent contributors to Barrett's Esophagus, several other factors are worth considering:

- **Age**: Barrett's Esophagus is more common in individuals over the age of 50, although it can occur at any age.

- **Gender**: Men are more commonly affected by Barrett's Esophagus than women, although the reasons for this gender disparity are not entirely understood.

- **Hiatal Hernia**: A hiatal hernia, where a portion of the stomach pushes through the diaphragm and into the chest, is associated with an increased risk of Barrett's Esophagus.

- **Ethnicity**: Some studies suggest that individuals of Caucasian descent are at a higher risk of developing Barrett's Esophagus compared to other ethnic groups.

Barrett's Esophagus is a multifactorial condition influenced by a combination of genetic predisposition, lifestyle choices, and underlying medical conditions. Understanding these causes and risk factors is crucial for identifying individuals at higher risk, implementing preventive measures, and guiding appropriate medical interventions to manage and monitor the condition effectively. Given its potential for progressing to esophageal cancer, an in-depth knowledge of these risk factors is paramount in ensuring the early detection and management of Barrett's Esophagus.

CHAPTER 3

Symptoms of Barrett's Esophagus

Barrett's Esophagus is a condition that often presents with subtle or no symptoms. However, it is crucial to be aware of potential signs, as it can progress to more serious conditions such as esophageal adenocarcinoma. we explore the various symptoms associated with Barrett's Esophagus, including heartburn and acid reflux, dysphagia (difficulty swallowing), chest pain, unexplained weight loss, and symptoms that may occur in advanced cases.

3.1 Heartburn and Acid Reflux

Heartburn and acid reflux are among the most common and recognizable symptoms of Barrett's Esophagus. Heartburn is described as a burning sensation or discomfort in the chest, often behind the breastbone, that can radiate up into the throat. This sensation is caused by the reflux of stomach acid into the esophagus. While occasional heartburn is common and usually harmless, frequent and persistent heartburn could be indicative of GERD, a significant risk factor for Barrett's Esophagus.

In Barrett's Esophagus, individuals may experience heartburn more frequently, and it may become more severe over time. It is important to note that not everyone with Barrett's

Esophagus experiences heartburn, and some individuals may have silent reflux, where stomach acid flows into the esophagus without causing noticeable symptoms.

3.2 Dysphagia (Difficulty Swallowing)

Dysphagia, or difficulty swallowing, is another symptom that individuals with Barrett's Esophagus may encounter. This symptom often develops as the condition progresses. The changes in the esophageal lining, including the development of scar tissue or strictures, can lead to narrowing of the esophagus. This narrowing can cause a sensation of food or liquids getting stuck in the throat or chest during swallowing.

Dysphagia can range from mild to severe, and it is more likely to occur with advanced stages of Barrett's Esophagus or when complications such as esophageal strictures are present. It is essential to address dysphagia promptly, as it can significantly impact an individual's quality of life and nutritional intake.

3.3 Chest Pain

Chest pain is another symptom that individuals with Barrett's Esophagus may experience. This pain can be similar to heartburn but is often more intense and may be mistaken for cardiac-related chest pain, especially in older individuals. It can be sharp, burning, or squeezing in nature and is typically felt behind the breastbone.

While chest pain associated with Barrett's Esophagus is usually related to acid reflux and irritation of the esophagus, it is essential not to dismiss chest pain without proper evaluation, as it can sometimes be challenging to distinguish from cardiac issues. Anyone experiencing new or severe chest pain should seek immediate medical attention.

3.4 Unexplained Weight Loss

Unexplained weight loss can be a concerning symptom associated with Barrett's Esophagus. Weight loss may occur due to various factors, including difficulty swallowing and decreased appetite, both of which can be consequences of advanced Barrett's Esophagus or its complications.

Significant and unintended weight loss should always be evaluated by a healthcare provider, as it can be indicative of underlying health issues, including the potential progression of Barrett's Esophagus to esophageal cancer. Timely medical assessment and intervention are crucial in such cases.

3.5 Symptoms in Advanced Cases

In advanced cases of Barrett's Esophagus, individuals may experience more severe and concerning symptoms, including:

- **Persistent vomiting**: Frequent vomiting or the presence of blood in vomit can be a sign of advanced complications, such as esophageal bleeding or obstruction.

- **Black or tarry stools**: Gastrointestinal bleeding, a potential complication of Barrett's Esophagus, can lead to the passage of black, tarry stools, which should be promptly reported to a healthcare provider.

- **Anemia**: Chronic bleeding or complications may result in anemia, leading to symptoms such as fatigue, weakness, and pallor.

- **Advanced difficulty swallowing**: Severe dysphagia can make it nearly impossible to swallow even liquids, posing a significant risk to nutritional intake.

It's crucial to emphasize that not everyone with Barrett's Esophagus will progress to advanced stages or experience severe symptoms. However, recognizing the symptoms associated with Barrett's Esophagus and seeking medical evaluation and management when necessary is vital to ensure early intervention and prevent potential complications, including esophageal cancer. Regular surveillance and monitoring are recommended for individuals with Barrett's Esophagus to detect any concerning changes in the esophageal lining early in its development.

CHAPTER 4

Diagnosis of Barrett's Esophagus

Diagnosing Barrett's Esophagus is a critical step in identifying and managing this condition, especially considering its potential for progression to esophageal adenocarcinoma. we explore the primary methods of diagnosis, including endoscopy and biopsy, imaging tests, and screening guidelines.

4.1 Endoscopy and Biopsy

Endoscopy is the gold standard for diagnosing Barrett's Esophagus. During an endoscopic examination, a thin, flexible tube with a light and camera (endoscope) is passed through the mouth and down the esophagus. This procedure allows healthcare providers to directly visualize the esophageal lining and identify any changes or abnormalities.

Biopsy is typically performed during endoscopy to confirm the diagnosis. During a biopsy, small tissue samples are collected from the affected area of the esophagus. These tissue samples are then examined under a microscope by a pathologist to determine whether the characteristic changes of Barrett's Esophagus, such as intestinal metaplasia, are present.

The biopsy results are crucial for confirming the diagnosis and grading the severity of Barrett's Esophagus. Grading helps in assessing the risk of progression to esophageal adenocarcinoma, with higher grades indicating a greater risk.

4.2 Imaging Tests

In addition to endoscopy and biopsy, imaging tests may be used to support the diagnosis of Barrett's Esophagus and assess the extent of the condition. These imaging modalities include:

- **Barium swallow**: This is a type of X-ray in which the patient drinks a contrast material containing barium. The barium coats the esophagus, making it visible on X-ray images. It can reveal structural abnormalities in the esophagus, such as strictures or irregularities in the lining.

- **Endoscopic ultrasound (EUS)**: EUS combines endoscopy with ultrasound to provide detailed images of the esophageal wall and surrounding structures. It is useful in evaluating the depth and extent of the condition, particularly in cases where cancer is suspected.

- **CT (computed tomography) scan**: CT scans can help assess the extent of Barrett's Esophagus and detect any abnormalities in nearby structures, such as lymph nodes.

These imaging tests are often used in conjunction with endoscopy to provide a comprehensive evaluation of the condition.

4.3 Screening Guidelines

Screening for Barrett's Esophagus is typically recommended for individuals who are at an elevated risk due to factors such as chronic GERD, family history of Barrett's Esophagus or esophageal cancer, or other risk factors. Screening guidelines may vary by region and healthcare provider, but common recommendations include:

- **Frequent or severe GERD**: Individuals with chronic or severe GERD symptoms, especially those who do not respond well to medication, are often considered candidates for screening.

- **Age and risk factors**: Screening may be recommended for individuals over the age of 50 with additional risk factors, such as obesity or a history of smoking.

- **Family history**: Individuals with a family history of Barrett's Esophagus or esophageal cancer may be advised to undergo screening.

- **Prior diagnosis of dysplasia**: If a person has been diagnosed with low-grade dysplasia or other concerning changes in the esophagus, regular surveillance through endoscopy may be recommended.

It's important to note that screening for Barrett's Esophagus should be conducted under the guidance of a healthcare provider, as it involves invasive procedures like endoscopy. The goal of screening is to detect the condition at an early stage, allowing for timely management and monitoring to reduce the risk of progression to esophageal adenocarcinoma.

The diagnosis of Barrett's Esophagus relies on a combination of methods, including endoscopy with biopsy, imaging tests, and adherence to screening guidelines. Timely and accurate diagnosis is essential for initiating appropriate treatment and surveillance measures, ultimately improving outcomes for individuals with this condition. Regular follow-up and adherence to recommended surveillance intervals are crucial to monitor any changes in the esophageal lining and manage the condition effectively.

CHAPTER 5

Grading and staging in Barrett's Esophagus

Grading and staging are essential aspects of evaluating Barrett's Esophagus, helping healthcare providers assess the severity of the condition and the associated cancer risk.

5.1 Stages of Barrett's Esophagus

Barrett's Esophagus is typically categorized into different stages based on the extent and characteristics of the

changes in the esophageal lining.
These stages include:

- **Non-dysplastic Barrett's Esophagus (NDBE)**: This stage represents the earliest form of Barrett's Esophagus. In NDBE, there are changes in the esophageal lining, but no evidence of dysplasia (abnormal cell growth). The risk of cancer in NDBE is relatively low, but surveillance is still recommended due to the potential for progression.

- **Low-grade dysplasia (LGD)**: Low-grade dysplasia is a stage where there are abnormal changes in the cells lining the esophagus, but these changes are considered mild. While the risk of cancer is still relatively low, individuals with LGD often undergo more frequent surveillance to monitor for any progression.

- **High-grade dysplasia (HGD)**: High-grade dysplasia is a more advanced stage where there are more significant and abnormal changes in the esophageal cells. HGD is associated with a higher risk of developing esophageal adenocarcinoma. It is considered a precancerous stage, and management options may include close surveillance or treatment.

- **Esophageal adenocarcinoma**: This is the most advanced stage and represents the development of cancer in the esophagus. Esophageal adenocarcinoma may develop in individuals with Barrett's Esophagus who have not received appropriate management or surveillance. Early detection and treatment of dysplasia can help prevent the progression to cancer.

It is crucial to understand that not all individuals with Barrett's Esophagus will progress to advanced stages or develop cancer. However, regular surveillance and monitoring are essential to detect any changes in the esophageal lining and initiate appropriate management when needed.

5.2 Dysplasia and Cancer Risk

Dysplasia is a critical factor in assessing the cancer risk associated with Barrett's Esophagus. Dysplasia refers to the abnormal growth and appearance of cells in the esophageal lining. It is typically categorized into two main types:

- **Low-grade dysplasia (LGD)**: In LGD, the changes in cell structure are relatively mild and do not show significant evidence of cancer development. However, LGD is still considered a precancerous condition, and individuals with LGD are at an increased risk of developing esophageal adenocarcinoma compared to those with non-dysplastic Barrett's Esophagus.

- **High-grade dysplasia (HGD)**: HGD represents more advanced and abnormal changes in cell structure and is associated with a higher risk of cancer development. HGD is considered a significant precancerous stage, and the risk of progression to esophageal adenocarcinoma is substantially higher than in LGD or non-dysplastic Barrett's Esophagus.

Dysplasia is typically identified through biopsies taken during endoscopic surveillance. The presence of dysplasia can influence the healthcare provider's recommendations for managing Barrett's Esophagus. This may include more frequent surveillance, endoscopic therapies to remove abnormal cells, or even surgical intervention in cases of HGD or advanced cancer.

grading and staging are crucial in assessing the severity and cancer risk associated with Barrett's Esophagus.

The presence of dysplasia, especially high-grade dysplasia, is a significant indicator of increased cancer risk, highlighting the importance of regular surveillance and timely intervention to prevent the progression of Barrett's Esophagus to esophageal adenocarcinoma. Early detection and management of dysplasia play a pivotal role in improving outcomes for individuals with this condition.

CHAPTER 6

Treatment Options

Barrett's Esophagus management involves a range of treatment options aimed at preventing the progression of the condition to esophageal adenocarcinoma, managing symptoms, and improving the patient's overall quality of life.

6.1 Lifestyle Modifications

Lifestyle modifications are often the first line of defense in managing Barrett's Esophagus, especially when it is associated with gastroesophageal reflux disease (GERD). These modifications can help reduce the frequency and severity of acid reflux, which is a significant contributor to the development and progression of Barrett's Esophagus. Key lifestyle changes include:

- **Dietary adjustments**: Avoiding trigger foods such as fatty, fried, spicy, and acidic foods can help minimize reflux symptoms. Consuming smaller, more frequent meals and avoiding late-night eating can also be beneficial.

- **Weight management**: Losing excess weight can reduce abdominal pressure, which can contribute to acid reflux. Maintaining a healthy weight through diet and exercise is recommended.

- **Elevating the head of the bed**: Raising the head of the bed by 6-8 inches can help prevent nighttime reflux symptoms.

- **Smoking cessation**: Quitting smoking can reduce the risk of weakening the lower esophageal sphincter, which can lead to increased acid reflux.

- **Limiting alcohol intake**: Alcohol can relax the lower esophageal sphincter, making it easier for stomach acid to flow back into the esophagus. Reducing alcohol consumption or avoiding it altogether may help manage symptoms.

- **Stress management**: High levels of stress can exacerbate GERD symptoms. Practicing stress-reduction techniques, such as mindfulness, yoga, or meditation, can be beneficial.

6.2 Medications

Medications are often prescribed to manage the symptoms of Barrett's Esophagus and reduce the acidity of stomach contents to prevent further damage to the esophageal lining. Commonly used medications include:

- **Proton pump inhibitors (PPIs)**: PPIs are powerful acid-reducing medications that are often prescribed to individuals with Barrett's Esophagus. They can help alleviate heartburn and reduce the risk of esophageal injury caused by acid reflux.

- **H2 blockers**: These medications reduce stomach acid production and can provide relief from heartburn and acid reflux symptoms.

- **Antacids**: Over-the-counter antacids can help neutralize stomach acid and provide temporary relief from heartburn.

- **Prokinetics**: Prokinetic medications can improve the motility of the esophagus and reduce the likelihood of acid reflux.

The choice of medication and its dosage may vary depending on the severity of symptoms and individual response to treatment. Healthcare providers will carefully assess and adjust medication regimens as needed.

6.3 Endoscopic Therapy

Endoscopic therapy is a treatment option used for individuals with Barrett's Esophagus who have dysplasia or other concerning changes in the esophageal lining. It aims to remove or treat abnormal cells and prevent the progression to esophageal adenocarcinoma. Common endoscopic therapies include:

- **Endoscopic mucosal resection (EMR)**: EMR involves the removal of abnormal tissue from the esophageal lining using an endoscope with specialized tools. It is typically used for the treatment of dysplasia.

- **Radiofrequency ablation (RFA)**: RFA uses controlled heat energy to destroy abnormal cells in the esophagus. It is effective in eliminating dysplasia and reducing the risk of cancer.

- **Cryotherapy**: Cryotherapy involves freezing and destroying abnormal tissue in the esophagus. It is another option for treating dysplasia.

- **Photodynamic therapy (PDT)**: PDT uses light-activated drugs to target and destroy abnormal cells. It is typically reserved for more advanced cases.

The choice of endoscopic therapy depends on the specific characteristics of the patient's Barrett's Esophagus and any associated dysplasia. Endoscopic therapies are less invasive than surgical interventions and can be highly effective in managing the condition.

The treatment of Barrett's Esophagus is tailored to the individual's specific circumstances, including the presence of dysplasia and the severity of symptoms. Lifestyle modifications, medications, and endoscopic therapy play crucial roles in managing the condition, preventing cancer progression, and improving the overall well-being of affected individuals. Regular follow-up and surveillance are essential components of Barrett's Esophagus management to monitor any changes in the esophageal lining and adjust treatment strategies accordingly.

6.4 Surgical Intervention

In some cases of Barrett's Esophagus, especially when there is a significant risk of cancer development, severe dysplasia, or when conservative treatments are ineffective, surgical intervention may be recommended. Surgery for Barrett's Esophagus typically aims to remove the affected tissue or prevent further reflux of stomach acid. Here are some common surgical options:

- **Fundoplication**: This procedure involves wrapping the top of the stomach around the lower esophagus to strengthen the lower esophageal sphincter, reducing the risk of acid reflux.

- **Esophagectomy**: In more advanced cases or when cancer

is present, a portion of the esophagus may need to be removed. The remaining portion of the esophagus is then connected to the stomach or another part of the digestive tract.

- **Laparoscopic anti-reflux surgery**: This minimally invasive procedure is used to reinforce the lower esophageal sphincter and prevent acid reflux. It may be considered when medications and lifestyle modifications are ineffective.

The choice of surgical intervention depends on the individual's specific condition and the recommendations of healthcare providers. Surgery is typically reserved for cases where the benefits outweigh the risks, as it carries potential complications and a longer recovery period compared to less invasive treatments.

6.5 Surveillance and Follow-up

Regular surveillance and follow-up are critical components of managing Barrett's Esophagus. Since Barrett's Esophagus is associated with an increased risk of esophageal adenocarcinoma, routine monitoring is essential for early detection and intervention. Here's what surveillance and follow-up entail:

- **Endoscopic surveillance**: Individuals with Barrett's Esophagus, particularly those with dysplasia, undergo regular endoscopic examinations (typically every 1-3 years) to assess the esophageal lining. During these endoscopies, tissue biopsies may be taken to check for changes in the cells.

- **Dysplasia management**: If dysplasia is detected during surveillance, healthcare providers may recommend more frequent follow-up endoscopies or endoscopic therapies to remove or treat abnormal cells.

- **Medication management**: Medications to manage acid reflux, such as proton pump inhibitors (PPIs) or H2 blockers, may be adjusted or continued as part of ongoing treatment.

- **Lifestyle counseling**: Patients are often counseled on lifestyle modifications to minimize reflux symptoms and reduce the risk of progression.

Surveillance and follow-up strategies are personalized based on the patient's specific risk factors, the presence of dysplasia, and the overall management plan. Timely and regular follow-up is crucial to detect any concerning changes in the esophageal lining and to adjust treatment strategies as needed.

surgical intervention is considered in specific cases of Barrett's Esophagus, especially when there is a high risk of cancer, severe dysplasia, or when conservative treatments are ineffective. Regular surveillance and follow-up are essential to monitor the condition, detect any abnormalities early, and ensure that the appropriate treatment and management strategies are in place. Early detection and intervention are key to improving outcomes and reducing the risk of esophageal adenocarcinoma in individuals with Barrett's Esophagus.

CHAPTER 7

Complications of Barrett's Esophagus

Barrett's Esophagus is associated with several potential complications, two of the most significant of which are esophageal adenocarcinoma and strictures. Understanding these complications is crucial for individuals with Barrett's Esophagus and their healthcare providers to monitor and manage the condition effectively.

7.1 Esophageal Adenocarcinoma

Esophageal adenocarcinoma is one of the most serious complications of Barrett's Esophagus. Individuals with Barrett's Esophagus are at an increased risk of developing esophageal cancer, and the risk is directly related to the presence and severity of dysplasia (abnormal cell growth) within the Barrett's tissue.

The progression from Barrett's Esophagus to esophageal adenocarcinoma typically occurs in stages, with non-dysplastic Barrett's Esophagus having a lower risk compared to low-grade dysplasia, high-grade dysplasia, and ultimately, cancer. Surveillance and regular endoscopic examinations are critical to detect dysplasia and early-stage cancer, as early intervention can lead to more favorable treatment outcomes.

Esophageal adenocarcinoma is a potentially life-threatening condition, and its treatment may involve surgery, chemotherapy, radiation therapy, or a combination of these approaches. Timely and regular surveillance is essential for detecting cancer at an early, potentially curable stage.

7.2 Strictures

Strictures in the esophagus are another common complication of Barrett's Esophagus. Strictures are characterized by the narrowing of the esophageal lumen, which can lead to difficulty swallowing (dysphagia) and discomfort.

Strictures can develop as a result of chronic irritation and inflammation of the esophageal lining due to acid reflux and the changes associated with Barrett's Esophagus. Scar tissue forms, causing the esophagus to become less elastic and more rigid.

Treatment for strictures may involve:

- **Endoscopic dilation**: In this procedure, a thin tube (dilator) is passed through an endoscope to gently stretch and widen the narrowed portion of the esophagus. Multiple dilation sessions may be required.

- **Medications**: Proton pump inhibitors (PPIs) and acid-suppressing medications may be prescribed to reduce inflammation and prevent further irritation.

- **Endoscopic therapies**:
  Endoscopic techniques, such as
  radiofrequency ablation (RFA)
  or cryotherapy, can be used to
  treat underlying Barrett's tissue
  and reduce the risk of strictures.

In severe cases where strictures do not
respond to less invasive treatments,
surgery may be necessary to remove
the narrowed portion of the esophagus
and reattach the remaining segments.

Strictures can significantly impact a
person's quality of life by making it
challenging to swallow and eat, so
prompt diagnosis and appropriate
management are crucial.

Barrett's Esophagus can lead to
several complications, with
esophageal adenocarcinoma and
strictures being among the most
significant. Regular surveillance,

early detection of dysplasia, and effective management of symptoms are key to minimizing the risk of these complications and improving the overall prognosis for individuals with Barrett's Esophagus.

CHAPTER 8

Prevention and Risk Reduction

Preventing Barrett's Esophagus and reducing the risk of its progression to esophageal adenocarcinoma primarily involve addressing risk factors and adopting healthy lifestyle practices. In this discussion, we explore two key strategies for prevention and risk reduction: managing gastroesophageal reflux disease (GERD) and weight management.

8.1 Managing GERD

Gastroesophageal reflux disease (GERD) is a major risk factor for the development of Barrett's Esophagus. Effective management of GERD can significantly reduce the risk of developing Barrett's Esophagus and its complications. Here are some strategies for managing GERD:

- **Medications**: Over-the-counter or prescription medications, such as proton pump inhibitors (PPIs) and H2 blockers, can help reduce stomach acid production and alleviate symptoms of GERD. These medications may be used as short-term relief or as long-term maintenance therapy, depending on the severity of symptoms.

- **Lifestyle modifications**: Making specific changes to your daily habits can help manage GERD. These include:

- **Dietary adjustments**: Avoid trigger foods that can exacerbate reflux symptoms, such as spicy, fatty, fried, and acidic foods. Smaller, more frequent meals can also help reduce the risk of reflux.

- **Elevating the head of the bed**: Raising the head of your bed by 6-8 inches can help prevent nighttime reflux symptoms.

- **Weight loss**: If you are overweight or obese, losing excess weight can reduce abdominal pressure, which can contribute to GERD. Maintaining a healthy weight through diet and exercise is recommended.

- **Smoking cessation**: Quitting smoking can help strengthen the lower esophageal sphincter and reduce the likelihood of acid reflux.

- **Stress management**: High levels of stress can exacerbate GERD symptoms. Practicing stress-reduction techniques, such as mindfulness, yoga, or meditation, can be beneficial.

8.2 Weight Management

Obesity is another significant risk factor for both GERD and Barrett's Esophagus. Managing your weight through a healthy lifestyle can help reduce the risk of developing these conditions. Here's how weight management can be achieved:

- **Dietary choices**: Adopting a balanced and nutritious diet can aid in weight management.

Focus on whole foods, fruits, vegetables, lean proteins, and whole grains while limiting processed and high-calorie foods.

- **Regular physical activity**: Engaging in regular exercise not only helps with weight management but can also reduce the risk of GERD by promoting healthy digestion. Aim for at least 150 minutes of moderate-intensity aerobic activity or 75 minutes of vigorous-intensity aerobic activity per week.

- **Portion control**: Be mindful of portion sizes to prevent overeating and excessive calorie intake.

- **Hydration**: Staying adequately hydrated is essential for overall health and can help control appetite.

- **Seeking support**: If weight management is challenging, consider working with a registered dietitian or healthcare provider to create a personalized plan.

By managing GERD and maintaining a healthy weight, you can significantly reduce the risk of developing Barrett's Esophagus and its complications. These lifestyle changes not only promote better digestive health but also contribute to overall well-being. If you have GERD or are at risk of Barrett's Esophagus due to family history or other factors, it's essential to work closely with your healthcare provider to develop a personalized prevention and risk reduction plan. Regular check-ups and screenings are also important for early detection and intervention if needed.

8.3 Lifestyle Changes

In addition to managing GERD and maintaining a healthy weight, several lifestyle changes can contribute to the prevention and risk reduction of Barrett's Esophagus. These changes aim to minimize the risk factors associated with the development and progression of the condition. Here are some important lifestyle modifications to consider:

- **Dietary modifications**: In addition to managing GERD-triggering foods, consider incorporating more fruits, vegetables, whole grains, and lean proteins into your diet. These foods are not only beneficial for weight management but also support overall digestive health.

- **Meal timing**: Avoid eating large meals close to bedtime, as lying down shortly after eating can increase the risk of acid reflux. Aim for a gap of at least two to three hours between your last meal and bedtime.

- **Avoiding tobacco and alcohol**: Quit smoking if you are a smoker, as tobacco use can weaken the lower esophageal sphincter and increase the risk of GERD. Reducing or eliminating alcohol consumption can also help manage GERD symptoms.

- **Staying upright after meals**: Remaining upright, whether it's standing or sitting, for at least two to three hours after eating can help prevent acid reflux by allowing gravity to assist in keeping stomach contents down.

- **Chewing gum**: Chewing sugarless gum after meals can stimulate saliva production, which can help neutralize stomach acid and reduce the risk of reflux.

- **Maintaining proper posture**: When sitting or standing, maintaining good posture can prevent added pressure on the abdomen, which can contribute to acid reflux.

- **Stress reduction**: Chronic stress can exacerbate GERD symptoms, so incorporating stress-reduction techniques into your daily routine, such as meditation, deep breathing exercises, or yoga, can be beneficial.

8.4 Regular Screening

Regular screening and surveillance are crucial components of preventing Barrett's Esophagus and managing its progression. Screening is typically recommended for individuals at an increased risk due to factors such as chronic GERD, family history of Barrett's Esophagus or esophageal cancer, or other risk factors.

Key aspects of regular screening and surveillance include:

- **Endoscopic examinations**: Regular endoscopic examinations are performed to assess the esophageal lining for any changes, such as the presence of Barrett's tissue or dysplasia. These exams are typically scheduled based on individual risk factors and healthcare provider recommendations.

- **Biopsy and tissue analysis**: During endoscopy, tissue samples (biopsies) may be collected and analyzed to detect any abnormal cells or changes in the esophageal lining.

- **Follow-up appointments**: Regular follow-up appointments with your healthcare provider ensure that any detected changes are monitored and managed promptly.

- **Adherence to screening guidelines**: It's essential to follow the recommended screening guidelines provided by your healthcare provider. These guidelines are tailored to your specific risk factors and the presence of Barrett's Esophagus.

Undergoing regular screening and surveillance, individuals at risk for Barrett's Esophagus can detect the condition at an early stage, enabling timely intervention and management. This proactive approach is critical for preventing the progression to esophageal adenocarcinoma, which is a potential complication of Barrett's Esophagus.

www.ingramcontent.com/pod-product-compliance
Lightning Source LLC
Chambersburg PA
CBHW062244290526
45794CB00006B/2401